NAVIGATING THE MIND: A COMPREHENSIVE GUIDE TO MENTAL HEALTH

BY OLUSEGUN AJULO

TABLE OF CONTENTS

INTRODUCTION

definition of mental health

Mental health refers to a person's emotional, psychological, and social well-being. It involves how individuals think, feel, and act as they face life's challenges, make choices, and relate to others. Mental health is crucial at every stage of life, from childhood and adolescence through adulthood. It affects how people handle stress, relate to others, and make decisions.

significance of mental health

1. Overall Well-Being: Mental health is essential for overall well-being. When individuals are mentally healthy, they can form positive relationships, work productively, cope with stress, and make meaningful contributions to society.

2. Emotional Stability: Good mental health enables individuals to manage their emotions effectively, fostering a sense of balance and stability in their lives. This emotional stability helps in navigating the ups and downs of life with resilience.

3. Physical Health: Mental health is interconnected with physical health. Poor mental health can negatively impact physical health, leading to issues like sleep disturbances, weakened immune system, and even chronic illnesses.

4. Quality of Life: Mental health significantly influences a person's quality of life. Positive mental health enhances one's ability to enjoy life, pursue goals, and experience a sense of fulfillment and purpose.

5. Productivity: Mental well-being is linked to productivity in various aspects of life, including work and education. Individuals with good mental health tend to be more focused, creative, and motivated, leading to increased productivity.

6. Healthy Relationships: Mental health plays a crucial role in forming and maintaining healthy relationships. It enables individuals to communicate effectively, empathize with others, and

establish meaningful connections, fostering positive interactions with family, friends, and colleagues.

7. Resilience: A mentally healthy individual is more resilient in the face of challenges and setbacks. They can bounce back from adversity, learn from experiences, and adapt to change effectively.

8. Reduced Stigma: Promoting mental health awareness reduces the stigma associated with mental illnesses. Understanding mental health encourages empathy, support, and acceptance for individuals experiencing mental health challenges, fostering a more compassionate society.

In summary, mental health is not just the absence of mental disorders; it encompasses emotional and social well-being, enabling individuals to lead fulfilling lives, maintain healthy relationships, and contribute meaningfully to their communities. Its significance lies in its profound impact on various aspects of life and the overall holistic health of individuals and societies.

importance of mental health awareness

1. Reduction of Stigma: Mental health awareness campaigns help reduce the stigma associated with mental illnesses. By promoting understanding and empathy, society becomes more accepting and supportive of individuals struggling with mental health challenges.

2. Early Intervention: Increased awareness leads to early recognition of mental health issues. Early intervention and treatment are vital in managing and overcoming many mental health conditions. Awareness campaigns encourage people to seek help promptly.

3. Prevention: Mental health awareness educates people about the risk factors and warning signs of mental illnesses. This knowledge empowers individuals to make lifestyle changes and seek support before problems escalate, potentially preventing the onset of severe conditions.

4. Improved Support Systems: When the general public, friends, and family members are aware of mental health issues, they can provide better support to those in need. This understanding fosters a more compassionate environment for individuals dealing with mental health challenges.

5. Enhanced Treatment Access: Awareness initiatives often highlight available mental health services and resources. This information can guide individuals to appropriate treatment options, ensuring they receive the help they need in a timely manner.

6. Promotion of Positive Mental Health: Mental health awareness is not just about addressing mental illnesses; it also emphasizes the importance of positive mental health and well-being. Understanding how to maintain good mental health promotes resilience, stress management, and overall life satisfaction.

7. Workplace Productivity: Mental health awareness in the workplace leads to better employee well-being. Employers can create supportive environments, offer counseling services, and implement stress-reduction programs. This, in turn, enhances employee productivity and job satisfaction.

8. Suicide Prevention: Mental health awareness campaigns often focus on suicide prevention. Educating the public about the signs of suicidal ideation and available crisis hotlines can save lives by enabling timely intervention and support.

9. Promoting Open Dialogue: Mental health awareness encourages open conversations about mental health. When people are comfortable discussing their struggles, it fosters a sense of community and reduces isolation, leading to better emotional health outcomes.

10. Societal Impact: By raising awareness about mental health, societies can address the economic and social impact of mental illnesses. This includes reducing healthcare costs, improving educational outcomes, and minimizing the burden on families and communities.

In summary, mental health awareness is vital for creating a compassionate and supportive society. It not only helps individuals in their personal struggles but also contributes to the overall well-being and productivity of communities. By understanding mental health issues, we can work together to create a more inclusive and empathetic world for everyone.

personal anecdotes or real-life examples illustrating mental health struggles

Here are a couple of real-life examples illustrating mental health struggles:

Example 1: Sarah's Battle with Anxiety

Sarah, a young professional, seemed confident and successful to her friends and colleagues. However, behind her cheerful facade, she battled crippling anxiety. The pressure to excel at work and maintain a perfect image took a toll on her mental health. She often found herself overwhelmed, experiencing panic attacks and sleepless nights. With the support of her friends and therapy, Sarah learned coping strategies and mindfulness techniques. Through her journey, she realized the importance of seeking help and speaking openly about mental health challenges.

Example 2: Mark's Experience with Depression

Mark, a college student, faced a severe bout of depression after a series of personal setbacks. He withdrew from social activities, lost interest in his hobbies, and struggled with daily tasks. Mark's friends and family noticed the change and encouraged him to seek professional help. With therapy and medication, Mark slowly began his recovery journey. It wasn't easy, but with time, he regained his enthusiasm for life. Mark's story highlights the transformative power of support, therapy, and resilience in overcoming depression.

These examples illustrate the real-life struggles individuals face with mental health issues and emphasize the importance of support, understanding, and seeking professional help in the recovery process.

UNDERSTANDING MENTAL HEALTH

Exploring common mental health disorders

1. Anxiety Disorders:

Anxiety disorders are characterized by excessive worry, fear, or apprehension. Common types include:

- Generalized Anxiety Disorder (GAD): Persistent and excessive worry about various aspects of life, even when there is little or no reason to worry.

- Panic Disorder: Recurrent, unexpected panic attacks accompanied by intense fear and physical symptoms like rapid heart rate and shortness of breath.

- Social Anxiety Disorder: Intense fear of social situations, leading to avoidance of social interactions and significant distress.

- Obsessive-Compulsive Disorder (OCD): Persistent, unwanted thoughts (obsessions) and repetitive behaviors or mental acts (compulsions) performed to reduce anxiety.

2. Depression:

Depression, also known as major depressive disorder, is a mood disorder that affects how a person feels, thinks, and handles daily activities. Symptoms include:

- Persistent sad, anxious, or "empty" mood

- Loss of interest or pleasure in activities once enjoyed

- Feelings of hopelessness or pessimism

- Changes in appetite or weight

- Sleep disturbances

- Fatigue or loss of energy

- Feelings of guilt or worthlessness

- Difficulty concentrating or making decisions

- Suicidal thoughts or attempts

3. Bipolar Disorder:

Bipolar disorder involves alternating periods of depression and mania (or hypomania). There are two main types:

- Bipolar I Disorder: Characterized by manic episodes that last at least seven days, or manic symptoms severe enough to require immediate hospitalization. Depressive episodes often occur as well.

- Bipolar II Disorder: Characterized by a pattern of depressive episodes and hypomanic episodes, which are less severe than full-blown manic episodes but still significantly impact daily functioning.

4. Post-Traumatic Stress Disorder (PTSD):

PTSD can develop after experiencing or witnessing a traumatic event. Symptoms may include:

- Flashbacks or intrusive memories of the trauma

- Nightmares

- Severe anxiety and emotional distress

- Avoidance of reminders of the trauma

- Negative changes in mood and thinking

- Hyperarousal, including irritability, difficulty sleeping, and being easily startled

5. Schizophrenia:

Schizophrenia is a severe mental disorder characterized by distorted thinking and awareness, including hallucinations and delusions. People with schizophrenia may also exhibit:

- Disorganized speech and behavior

- Impaired cognitive functioning

- Social withdrawal and lack of motivation

- Difficulty in distinguishing between what is real and what is not

factors contributing to mental health issues

Understanding these common mental health disorders is crucial for early recognition, diagnosis, and appropriate treatment, leading to improved quality of life for individuals affected by these conditions.

1. Genetics:

Genetic factors play a significant role in the development of mental health issues. Certain mental disorders, such as schizophrenia, bipolar disorder, and some types of depression and anxiety disorders, tend to run in families. Having a close relative with a mental health disorder can increase an individual's risk of developing a similar condition due to shared genetic vulnerabilities.

2. Environmental Factors:

- Early Life Experiences: Adverse childhood experiences (ACEs), such as abuse, neglect, or dysfunctional family environments, can have a profound impact on mental health. Traumatic experiences during childhood can increase the risk of various mental health disorders later in life.

- Stressful Life Events: Chronic stress, major life changes, financial difficulties, or relationship problems can trigger or exacerbate mental health issues. High-stress levels can disrupt brain chemistry and contribute to the development of disorders like anxiety and depression.

- Social Isolation: Lack of social support and feelings of loneliness can negatively affect mental well-being. Social connections and supportive relationships are essential for emotional health and resilience.

3. Trauma:

- Physical or Emotional Trauma: Traumatic events, such as accidents, assaults, natural disasters, or witnessing violence, can lead to post-traumatic stress disorder (PTSD) and other mental health disorders. Emotional trauma, like a sudden loss or betrayal, can also have lasting psychological effects.

- Developmental Trauma: Trauma experienced during critical stages of development, particularly in childhood, can disrupt normal emotional and psychological growth. This disruption can manifest as various mental health challenges in adulthood.

4. Neurobiological Factors:

- Brain Chemistry: Imbalances in neurotransmitters (chemical messengers in the brain) like serotonin, dopamine, and norepinephrine are associated with mood disorders such as depression and bipolar disorder.

- Brain Structure: Structural abnormalities in certain brain regions have been observed in individuals with mental health disorders. For instance, differences in the amygdala and hippocampus are linked to anxiety and PTSD.

5. Substance Abuse:

Substance abuse, including alcohol and drugs, can worsen or trigger mental health issues. Substance use can disrupt brain function, exacerbate symptoms of existing mental disorders, or create new mental health problems.

Understanding the complex interplay of genetic, environmental, and trauma-related factors is crucial for mental health professionals to provide effective treatment and support. Early intervention, therapy, and a supportive environment can mitigate the impact of these factors and help individuals manage and overcome mental health challenges.

the stigma surrounding mental health and its impact

1. Social Isolation: Stigma often leads to social isolation and discrimination against individuals with mental health issues. People may avoid those who are open about their struggles, leading to feelings of loneliness and further exacerbating their mental health conditions.

2. Barriers to Seeking Help: Stigma creates barriers that prevent people from seeking mental health support. Fear of judgment and discrimination can deter individuals from reaching out to mental health professionals, friends, or family members for assistance. Consequently, they may avoid necessary treatment and suffer in silence.

3. Underdiagnosis and Misdiagnosis: Stigmatizing attitudes can influence healthcare professionals, leading to underdiagnosis or misdiagnosis of mental health disorders. Patients may not receive proper assessments or treatments due to biases, affecting their overall well-being.

4. Impact on Self-Esteem: Individuals facing stigma often internalize negative beliefs about themselves. This can significantly impact their self-esteem and self-worth, leading to diminished confidence and increased vulnerability to mental health issues.

5. Employment Discrimination: Stigma can affect job opportunities and workplace environments. Individuals open about their mental health struggles might face discrimination in hiring or promotions. Fear of workplace discrimination often prevents employees from disclosing their conditions and seeking necessary accommodations.

6. Impact on Relationships: Stigmatization can strain relationships with friends, family, and romantic partners. Misunderstanding and prejudice can lead to strained interactions and broken connections, further isolating individuals from their support networks.

7. Treatment Disparities: Stigma contributes to disparities in mental health treatment. Certain communities, such as minorities or LGBTQ+ individuals, might face additional stigma, making it even harder to access appropriate and culturally competent mental health services.

8. Impact on Policy and Funding: Stigma can influence public policies and funding for mental health services. Societies with stigmatizing attitudes may not prioritize mental health funding, leading to limited resources and inadequate support systems for those in need.

9. Cycle of Shame: Stigmatizing attitudes perpetuate a cycle of shame and silence. When individuals feel ashamed or embarrassed about their mental health struggles, they are less likely to talk openly about their experiences, hindering collective efforts to combat stigma.

10. Preventing Timely Intervention: Stigma often delays intervention. People may wait until their conditions worsen significantly before seeking help, making treatment more challenging and reducing the likelihood of successful recovery.

Mental Health Across the Lifespan

Addressing mental health stigma is crucial for fostering a supportive environment where individuals feel safe to seek help, talk openly about their experiences, and access the resources they need. Public awareness campaigns, education, and promoting understanding are essential steps toward breaking down the barriers created by mental health stigma.

Childhood and Adolescent Mental Health Challenges:

1. Anxiety Disorders: Anxiety disorders, including generalized anxiety disorder and social anxiety disorder, are common among children and adolescents. Excessive worry, fear, and avoidance of social situations can significantly impact their daily lives and academic performance.

2. Depression: Childhood and adolescent depression can manifest as persistent sadness, lack of interest in activities, changes in sleep and appetite, and feelings of hopelessness. Untreated depression can interfere with academic achievements and social relationships.

3. Attention-Deficit/Hyperactivity Disorder (ADHD): ADHD is characterized by inattention, hyperactivity, and impulsivity. Children with ADHD may struggle with focusing on tasks, sitting still, and following instructions, leading to difficulties in school and conflicts with peers.

4. Autism Spectrum Disorders (ASD): ASD encompasses a range of developmental disorders affecting communication, behavior, and social interaction. Children with ASD may face challenges in social interactions, communication, and repetitive behaviors. Early intervention and therapy are crucial for improving outcomes.

5. Eating Disorders: Disorders like anorexia nervosa, bulimia nervosa, and binge-eating disorder can affect adolescents, particularly girls. These conditions involve unhealthy attitudes toward food, body weight, and shape, leading to severe physical and emotional consequences.

6. Self-Harm and Suicide: Some adolescents may engage in self-harm behaviors, such as cutting, burning, or excessive risk-taking. Untreated mental health issues and peer pressure can contribute to self-harm. In severe cases, untreated mental health challenges can lead to suicidal thoughts and attempts.

7. Obsessive-Compulsive Disorder (OCD): OCD in children and adolescents involves persistent, unwanted thoughts (obsessions) and repetitive behaviors or mental acts (compulsions). These rituals can significantly disrupt daily life and cause distress.

8. Post-Traumatic Stress Disorder (PTSD): Children and adolescents who experience trauma, such as abuse, violence, or natural disasters, can develop PTSD. Symptoms include flashbacks, nightmares, severe anxiety, and emotional numbness, affecting their overall well-being and ability to function.

9. Behavioral Disorders: Conduct disorder and oppositional defiant disorder are behavioral disorders characterized by persistent patterns of aggressive, defiant, or antisocial behavior. These challenges can lead to conflicts at home, school, and within the community.

10. Substance Abuse: Adolescents may turn to substance abuse as a way to cope with their mental health challenges. Substance abuse can exacerbate existing mental health conditions and lead to additional problems, such as academic difficulties and legal issues.

Early intervention, supportive family environments, access to mental health services, and school-based programs are crucial in addressing childhood and adolescent mental health challenges. Identifying symptoms early and providing appropriate treatment and support can significantly improve the outcomes and quality of life for young individuals facing these issues.

Adult mental health concerns

1. Work-Related Stress:

Work-related stress is a common adult mental health concern. High-pressure environments, tight deadlines, long working hours, and job insecurity can lead to chronic stress. Persistent stress at work may result in burnout, anxiety, and even depression. It can also impair decision-making abilities and overall job performance.

2. Relationship Issues:

Difficulties in relationships, whether with partners, family members, or friends, can significantly impact mental health. Conflict, communication breakdowns, and feelings of isolation or loneliness can lead to stress, anxiety, and depression. Relationship problems often contribute to emotional distress and may require therapy or counseling to resolve.

3. Marital or Partnership Strain:

Marital or partnership issues, including disagreements, financial stress, infidelity, or lack of intimacy, can lead to emotional turmoil. Unresolved problems in relationships can cause persistent worry, sadness, and feelings of hopelessness, affecting both partners' mental well-being.

4. Grief and Loss:

Coping with the loss of a loved one through death, divorce, or separation is a significant adult mental health concern. Grief can trigger intense emotions, such as sadness, anger, guilt, and profound sadness. Unresolved grief can lead to complicated grief reactions and may require therapeutic support.

5. Financial Stress:

Financial difficulties, such as debt, job loss, or the inability to meet basic needs, can cause significant stress and anxiety. Constant worry about finances can lead to sleep disturbances, low self-esteem, and strained relationships within families.

6. Parenting Challenges:

Parenting challenges, including parenting a child with special needs, dealing with behavioral issues, or managing the demands of balancing work and family life, can lead to parental stress. Feelings of inadequacy, frustration, and exhaustion are common concerns among parents, impacting their mental health.

7. Trauma and Abuse:

Adults who have experienced trauma, abuse, or violence, whether in childhood or later in life, may suffer from post-traumatic stress disorder (PTSD) or other mental health conditions. Traumatic experiences can lead to flashbacks, nightmares, and emotional distress, affecting daily functioning and relationships.

8. Chronic Health Conditions:

Managing chronic health conditions, such as diabetes, chronic pain, or autoimmune disorders, can cause emotional strain. Dealing with the challenges of ongoing medical treatments, pain, and lifestyle adjustments can lead to anxiety, depression, and reduced quality of life.

Addressing these adult mental health concerns often requires a combination of therapy, counseling, social support, and lifestyle changes. Seeking professional help and fostering strong social connections are essential steps toward managing and overcoming these challenges.

Mental health issues in the elderly population

Mental health issues in the elderly population are a significant concern, often overlooked. Conditions like depression, anxiety, and dementia are common. Social isolation, loss of loved ones, and physical health problems can contribute. It's crucial to raise awareness, offer support, and promote mental well-being in older adults through social connections, therapy, and appropriate healthcare.

SEEKING HELP

Recognizing signs of mental health problems

Recognizing signs of mental health problems can vary depending on the specific condition, but common signs include changes in mood, behavior, or thinking patterns. Look for withdrawal from social activities, drastic mood swings, persistent sadness, excessive worries, changes in sleep or appetite, and difficulty concentrating. Physical symptoms like unexplained aches or pains can also be related to mental health issues. If you notice these signs persisting, it's important to encourage the person to seek professional help from a mental health provider.

How to approach someone you suspect is struggling

Approaching someone you suspect is struggling with their mental health requires empathy, sensitivity, and understanding. Here are some steps you can take:

1. Choose the Right Time and Place: Find a quiet and comfortable setting where both of you can talk openly without distractions.

2. Be Empathetic and Non-Judgmental: Approach the person with kindness and understanding. Avoid being critical or judgmental about their feelings or experiences.

3. Listen Actively: Allow them to express their feelings and thoughts. Be an active listener, showing that you genuinely care about what they are saying.

4. Express Concern: Express your concern for their well-being. Use "I" statements to avoid sounding accusatory, such as "I've noticed you seem down lately, and I'm concerned about you."

5. Offer Support: Let them know that you are there for them and willing to help. Offer your support and encouragement for them to seek professional help if needed.

6. Encourage Professional Help: Suggest seeing a mental health professional, such as a therapist or counselor. Offer to help them find resources or accompany them to appointments if they are comfortable with that.

7. Respect Their Boundaries: Be respectful if they are not ready to talk or seek help immediately. Give them space but continue to check in and offer your support.

8. Follow Up: Check in on them regularly. A simple message or call can show that you still care and are there to support them.

Remember, you are not responsible for fixing their problems, but your support and understanding can make a significant difference.

Types of mental health professionals and their roles (psychiatrists, psychologists, counselors)

There are various types of mental health professionals, each with specific roles and expertise. Here are some common types:

1. Psychiatrist: A medical doctor who specializes in the diagnosis, treatment, and prevention of mental illnesses. They can prescribe medications and provide therapy.

2. Psychologist: Holds a doctoral degree in psychology (Ph.D. or Psy.D.) and provides therapy, counseling, and psychological testing. Psychologists cannot prescribe medications.

3. Licensed Professional Counselor (LPC) or Licensed Mental Health Counselor (LMHC): Trained to diagnose and provide therapy for individuals, couples, and families. They often work with issues like anxiety, depression, and relationships.

4. Clinical Social Worker (LCSW): Licensed to diagnose and treat mental health disorders. They provide therapy, support, and help clients navigate social services.

5. Psychotherapist: A general term for professionals who provide talk therapy to address emotional and mental health issues. This can include psychologists, counselors, social workers, and therapists.

6. Licensed Marriage and Family Therapist (LMFT): Specializes in working with couples and families to address relationship issues and family dynamics.

7. Psychiatric Nurse Practitioner (PMHNP): A nurse practitioner with specialized training in mental health. They can diagnose, provide therapy, and prescribe medications.

8. Counseling Psychologist: Focuses on helping people cope with everyday issues and life challenges. They often work in educational or research settings.

9. Art Therapist, Music Therapist, Drama Therapist: These professionals use creative arts as a form of therapy to help individuals express themselves and address emotional issues.

10. Occupational Therapist (OT): Helps people develop or regain the skills needed for daily living and working through therapeutic activities.

Remember, the specific roles and scopes of practice can vary based on the professional's credentials and the regulations in their region. It's essential to choose a professional based on your specific needs and their expertise.

TREATMENT AND COPING STRATEGIES

Therapy options

Certainly, there are various therapy options available to address different mental health concerns. Here are some common types of therapy:

1. Cognitive Behavioral Therapy (CBT): Focuses on identifying and changing negative thought patterns and behaviors to promote healthier ways of thinking and coping.

2. Psychodynamic Therapy: Explores unconscious thoughts and feelings to understand how past experiences influence present behavior, thoughts, and emotions.

3. Mindfulness-Based Therapies: Such as Mindfulness-Based Stress Reduction (MBSR) and Mindfulness-Based Cognitive Therapy (MBCT), which incorporate mindfulness practices to help individuals manage stress, anxiety, and depression.

4. Dialectical Behavior Therapy (DBT): Combines cognitive-behavioral techniques with mindfulness strategies to help individuals manage intense emotions, improve relationships, and develop coping skills.

5. Interpersonal Therapy (IPT): Focuses on improving communication and interpersonal skills to help individuals address relationship issues and manage mood disorders.

6. Exposure Therapy: Commonly used for anxiety disorders, it involves gradually facing feared situations or memories to reduce anxiety and fear responses.

7. Family Therapy: Involves working with families to improve communication, resolve conflicts, and address family dynamics that may contribute to mental health issues.

8. Group Therapy: Conducted in a group setting, it provides a supportive environment where individuals with similar concerns can share experiences, offer support, and learn coping skills from one another.

9. Trauma-Focused Therapy: Specifically designed to help individuals overcome the emotional and psychological effects of trauma through specialized techniques and interventions.

10. Art Therapy: Utilizes creative expression to help individuals explore and process their emotions, often beneficial for people who find it challenging to express themselves verbally.

11. Play Therapy: Primarily used with children, it allows them to communicate and express their feelings through play, toys, and other creative activities.

It's important to note that the effectiveness of therapy can vary depending on the individual and their specific needs. It's often helpful to consult with a mental health professional who can assess the situation and recommend an appropriate therapy approach tailored to the individual's concerns. Additionally, some individuals may benefit from a combination of therapies or therapies along with medication, depending on the severity of their condition.

Medications and their role in mental health treatment

Medications can play a crucial role in the treatment of mental health conditions. They are often prescribed to help manage symptoms and improve the overall quality of life for individuals with various mental health disorders. Here are common types of medications and their roles in mental health treatment:

1. Antidepressants: These medications are used to treat depression, anxiety disorders, and some other conditions. They work by balancing chemicals in the brain, particularly neurotransmitters like serotonin and norepinephrine, which influence mood.

2. Antianxiety Medications (Anxiolytics): These medications are prescribed to reduce symptoms of anxiety and excessive worry. They can help individuals feel calmer and reduce physical symptoms associated with anxiety disorders.

3. Antipsychotic Medications: Primarily used to manage symptoms of psychotic disorders like schizophrenia and bipolar disorder. They help control distorted thinking and perceptions, such as hallucinations or delusions.

4. Mood Stabilizers: Used to manage mood swings in bipolar disorder and related conditions. They help stabilize and maintain a normal mood, preventing episodes of mania or depression.

5. Stimulants: Often prescribed to treat attention-deficit/hyperactivity disorder (ADHD) by increasing dopamine and norepinephrine levels in the brain, which improves focus, attention, and impulse control.

6. Sedatives/Hypnotics: Prescribed for sleep disorders or severe anxiety. They help induce sleep and relaxation, and they are typically used on a short-term basis.

7. Opioid Medications: Sometimes used for severe pain management. However, due to their addictive nature, they require careful monitoring and should only be used as prescribed.

It's important to note that medication is not always the first line of treatment, and the decision to prescribe medication is made after a thorough evaluation by a healthcare professional. Mental health professionals consider factors such as the type and severity of the condition, the individual's overall health, and their response to other forms of treatment.

Additionally, medication is often most effective when combined with therapy and other non-pharmacological treatments. Regular follow-ups with a healthcare provider are essential to monitor the medication's effectiveness, adjust dosages if necessary, and manage potential side effects. It's crucial for individuals to communicate openly with their healthcare provider about their experiences and any concerns they may have while taking mental health medications.

Alternative therapies (mindfulness, meditation, yoga)

Alternative therapies like mindfulness, meditation, and yoga can be valuable complements to traditional mental health treatments. Here's how they can help:

1. Mindfulness: Mindfulness involves paying full attention to the present moment without judgment. It can reduce stress, enhance emotional regulation, and improve overall well-being. Practicing mindfulness can help individuals become more aware of their thoughts and feelings, allowing them to respond to situations in a calmer manner.

2. Meditation: Meditation techniques vary, but they often involve focusing the mind and eliminating the stream of jumbled thoughts. Regular meditation practice can promote relaxation, improve concentration, and reduce symptoms of anxiety and depression. It can also enhance self-awareness and lead to a greater sense of inner peace.

3. Yoga: Yoga combines physical postures, breathing exercises, and meditation. It can enhance flexibility, strength, and balance while promoting relaxation and stress reduction. Yoga's emphasis on mindfulness and breathing techniques can help individuals become more aware of their bodies and reduce symptoms of anxiety and depression.

These alternative therapies are often used in conjunction with traditional mental health treatments and can be tailored to an individual's specific needs. Many studies suggest that incorporating mindfulness, meditation, or yoga into one's routine can have positive effects on mental health, promoting a sense of calm and improving overall psychological well-being.

It's essential, however, to learn these practices from qualified instructors, especially if you're dealing with specific mental health concerns. Additionally, it's important to recognize that while these practices can be beneficial, they might not be a replacement for professional mental health treatment when needed. Consulting with a mental health professional can help determine the most suitable approach for individual circumstances.

developing healthy coping mechanisms

Developing healthy coping mechanisms is crucial for maintaining good mental health. Here are some strategies to consider:

1. Physical Activity: Regular exercise can boost your mood and reduce stress. It doesn't have to be intense – even a daily walk can make a difference.

2. Mindfulness and Meditation: Practicing mindfulness and meditation can help you stay present and manage negative thoughts and emotions.

3. Healthy Eating: A balanced diet can have a significant impact on your mood and energy levels. Avoid excessive caffeine, sugar, and processed foods.

4. Adequate Sleep: Getting enough sleep is essential for your overall well-being. Establish a regular sleep schedule and create a relaxing bedtime routine.

5. Social Support: Maintain strong connections with friends and family. Talking to someone you trust about your feelings can provide relief and support.

6. Limit Stressors: Identify sources of stress in your life and find ways to minimize or eliminate them. This could involve setting boundaries, saying no when necessary, or seeking professional help.

7. Creative Outlets: Engage in activities that allow you to express yourself, such as art, music, writing, or any other creative pursuit.

8. Hobbies and Interests: Pursue activities that bring you joy and a sense of accomplishment. Engaging in hobbies can provide a healthy distraction from negative thoughts.

9. Therapy and Counseling: Speaking to a mental health professional can provide you with coping strategies tailored to your specific situation.

10. Self-Compassion: Be kind and understanding to yourself, especially during difficult times. Treat yourself with the same compassion you would offer to a friend.

BUILDING RESILIENCE

Remember, finding the right coping mechanisms may take time and experimentation. It's essential to be patient with yourself and seek help if you need it.

Importance of self-care

Building resilience is crucial for navigating life's challenges, and self-care plays a central role in this process. Here's why self-care is important in fostering resilience:

1. Emotional Well-being: Self-care activities, such as mindfulness and relaxation techniques, help regulate emotions and reduce stress. By managing your emotions, you can approach challenges with a clearer and calmer mindset.

2. Physical Health: Regular exercise, proper nutrition, and sufficient sleep are fundamental aspects of self-care. When you take care of your body, you enhance your overall health and energy levels, making it easier to cope with stressors.

3. Self-Compassion: Self-care involves treating yourself with kindness and understanding, especially during difficult times. Developing self-compassion allows you to bounce back from setbacks and failures with a positive attitude.

4. Boundaries: Setting and maintaining boundaries is a form of self-care. It helps you protect your time, energy, and emotional well-being. Resilient individuals know when to say no and prioritize their own needs.

5. Problem-Solving Skills: Engaging in self-care activities provides time for reflection and introspection. This can enhance your problem-solving skills and help you develop a proactive approach to challenges.

6. Social Support: Self-care includes nurturing your relationships and seeking support when needed. Strong social connections act as a buffer against stress and provide a sense of belonging and security.

7. Preventing Burnout: Regular self-care prevents burnout, which can occur when you consistently neglect your own needs while taking care of others or dealing with challenging situations. Resilient individuals recognize the signs of burnout and take steps to prevent it.

8. Increased Confidence: Engaging in self-care activities that promote self-improvement, such as learning new skills or pursuing hobbies, can boost your confidence and self-esteem. This increased self-assurance helps you face adversity with a positive mindset.

9. Adaptability: Resilience is about adapting to change and bouncing back from setbacks. Engaging in self-care routines provides stability and a sense of routine, which can be especially helpful during times of change and uncertainty.

In essence, self-care is not selfish; it's a fundamental aspect of building resilience. By taking care of your physical, emotional, and mental well-being, you equip yourself with the strength and resources needed to face life's challenges with grace and determination.

Enhancing emotional intelligence

Enhancing emotional intelligence (EI) can greatly improve your interpersonal relationships, communication skills, and overall well-being. Here are some strategies to enhance your emotional intelligence:

1. Self-awareness: Pay attention to your emotions without judgment. Recognize how you're feeling and understand the reasons behind your emotions. Journaling can be helpful for self-reflection.

2. Self-regulation: Learn to manage your emotions effectively. Practice relaxation techniques, mindfulness, or deep breathing to stay calm in challenging situations. Avoid impulsive reactions and think before you respond.

3. Empathy: Put yourself in others' shoes. Practice active listening to understand others' perspectives. Show genuine interest in their feelings and experiences. Empathetic responses build stronger connections with others.

4. Social Skills: Develop strong communication skills. Be clear and concise in your speech. Work on your non-verbal cues, such as facial expressions and body language, to convey your emotions effectively. Practice conflict resolution and negotiation skills.

5. Motivation: Set and work towards meaningful goals. Find your passions and pursue them. Stay optimistic and resilient in the face of setbacks. A positive attitude can enhance your motivation and drive to succeed.

6. Practice Mindfulness: Regular mindfulness meditation can increase your awareness of emotions, thoughts, and bodily sensations. This awareness can help you respond more thoughtfully to situations rather than reacting impulsively.

7. Continuous Learning: Read books, attend workshops, or take courses on emotional intelligence. Educate yourself about different emotions, their triggers, and healthy ways to manage them.

8. Cultivate Empathetic Responses: When interacting with others, try to understand their emotions and respond with empathy. Acknowledge their feelings, even if you don't agree with them. Validation can go a long way in building trust and understanding.

9. Seek Feedback: Ask for feedback from trusted friends, family, or colleagues about your emotional intelligence. Constructive feedback can help you identify areas for improvement.

10. Practice Gratitude: Cultivating a sense of gratitude can enhance your emotional well-being. Regularly reflect on the things you're thankful for, even in challenging situations. Gratitude helps shift focus from negativity to positivity.

Remember, developing emotional intelligence is a continuous process that takes time and effort. Be patient with yourself and celebrate your progress along the way.

Building a supportive social network

Building a supportive social network is vital for your well-being and can provide a strong foundation for emotional support, companionship, and personal growth. Here are some strategies to help you build and maintain a supportive social network:

1. Identify Your Needs: Determine the type of support you need, whether it's emotional, practical, or social. Understanding your needs will guide you in seeking out the right kind of connections.

2. Be Open and Approachable: Approach social situations with an open and positive attitude. Smile, make eye contact, and be genuinely interested in others. Approach potential friendships with kindness and sincerity.

3. Join Communities: Participate in clubs, classes, sports teams, religious or spiritual groups, or hobbyist communities. Shared interests provide a natural platform for building connections.

4. Volunteer: Volunteering for charitable organizations or community events not only helps others but also allows you to meet like-minded individuals who are also passionate about making a difference.

5. Attend Social Events: Attend parties, gatherings, and community events even if you're shy or introverted. These events provide opportunities to meet new people in a relaxed atmosphere.

6. Stay Connected: Make an effort to stay in touch with existing friends and acquaintances. Regular communication, even if it's a quick message or call, strengthens relationships.

7. Be a Good Listener: Show genuine interest in others. Listen actively, ask open-ended questions, and validate their feelings. Being a good listener fosters trust and deepens connections.

8. Offer Support: Be supportive and helpful to others in your network. Acts of kindness and support create a reciprocal atmosphere where others are more likely to be supportive in return.

9. Set Boundaries: While it's essential to be supportive, it's also crucial to set boundaries. Be mindful of your own well-being and avoid relationships that are consistently negative or draining.

10. Online Communities: Participate in online forums, social media groups, or support communities related to your interests. These platforms can provide a sense of belonging and connect you with people who share your passions.

11. Attend Workshops and Classes: Enroll in workshops or classes related to your hobbies or interests. Not only do you learn something new, but you also have the opportunity to meet people who share your enthusiasm.

Remember, building a supportive social network takes time and effort. Be patient, be genuine, and invest in the relationships that bring positivity and support into your life.

Managing stress and adversity effectively

Managing stress and adversity effectively is essential for maintaining good mental and physical health. Here are strategies to help you cope with stress and overcome adversity:

1. Self-Care: Prioritize self-care activities, such as exercise, adequate sleep, and healthy nutrition. When you take care of your body, you're better equipped to handle stress.

2. Mindfulness and Relaxation: Practice mindfulness meditation, deep breathing exercises, or yoga. These techniques can help you stay present, reduce anxiety, and improve your overall well-being.

3. Positive Mindset: Cultivate a positive outlook on life. Focus on what you can control, and try to reframe negative thoughts into more positive and realistic ones.

4. Time Management: Organize your tasks and prioritize them. Break tasks into smaller, manageable steps, and set realistic goals. Effective time management can reduce feelings of being overwhelmed.

5. Social Support: Lean on your supportive social network—friends, family, or support groups. Talking to others about your feelings can provide emotional relief and different perspectives on the situation.

6. Problem-Solving: Identify the root cause of your stress and work on finding practical solutions. Brainstorm possible solutions, weigh their pros and cons, and take action.

7. Physical Activity: Regular exercise not only benefits your physical health but also releases endorphins, which are natural stress relievers. Aim for activities you enjoy, whether it's walking, dancing, or any other form of exercise.

8. Creative Outlets: Engage in creative activities that allow you to express your emotions, such as writing, painting, or playing a musical instrument. Creative expression can serve as a therapeutic outlet.

9. Seek Professional Help: If stress and adversity become overwhelming, don't hesitate to seek help from a therapist, counselor, or mental health professional. They can provide guidance and support tailored to your specific situation.

10. Practice Gratitude: Focus on the positive aspects of your life. Regularly expressing gratitude for the things, you have can shift your focus from what's stressful to what's meaningful and good in your life.

11. Learn to Say No: Set boundaries and don't overcommit yourself. It's okay to say no to additional responsibilities if you already have a lot on your plate.

12. Acceptance: Sometimes, situations are beyond our control. Practice acceptance of the things you cannot change. Acknowledge your feelings about the situation, and work on adapting to the new circumstances.

Remember that everyone faces challenges, and it's okay to ask for help when needed. By incorporating these strategies into your life, you can effectively manage stress and navigate adversity with resilience.

MENTAL HEALTH AND SOCIETY

Mental health policies and their impact on society

Mental health policies play a crucial role in shaping society by influencing access to care, reducing stigma, and promoting overall well-being. When well-implemented, these policies can have several positive impacts on society:

1. Improved Access to Treatment: Policies that prioritize mental health can lead to increased access to mental health services, ensuring that individuals receive timely and appropriate care.

2. Reduced Stigma: Public policies can contribute to reducing the stigma associated with mental health issues, encouraging more people to seek help without fear of discrimination or judgment.

3. Enhanced Productivity: By supporting mental health in the workplace, policies can enhance productivity as employees are better able to manage their mental health conditions, leading to reduced absenteeism and improved job satisfaction.

4. Prevention and Early Intervention: Policies that focus on prevention and early intervention can identify mental health issues in their early stages, preventing them from escalating into more serious conditions. This can lead to cost savings in the long run.

5. Family and Community Well-being: Mental health policies that support families and communities can strengthen social bonds and improve overall community well-being. This can lead to safer and more supportive environments for everyone.

6. Reduction in Crime and Substance Abuse: Adequate mental health support can reduce the likelihood of individuals engaging in criminal activities or substance abuse as coping mechanisms, contributing to overall community safety.

7. Positive Impact on Physical Health: Mental health policies can also have a positive impact on physical health outcomes, as mental and physical health are interconnected. Improved mental health can lead to healthier lifestyles and better management of chronic illnesses.

8. Educational Attainment: Mental health support in educational settings can enhance students' emotional well-being, leading to better focus, improved academic performance, and higher educational attainment rates.

9. Social Inclusion: Mental health policies that promote inclusion and equality can create a more compassionate society where individuals with mental health challenges are integrated into various aspects of community life.

Addressing mental health in workplaces and schools

It's important for societies to advocate for and implement comprehensive mental health policies that address the diverse needs of their populations, ensuring that mental health is treated with the same importance as physical health.

Addressing mental health in workplaces and schools is crucial for creating supportive environments where individuals can thrive. Here are some strategies that can be implemented in both settings:

In Workplaces:

1. Mental Health Programs: Implement workplace mental health programs that include counseling services, stress management workshops, and awareness campaigns. Encourage employees to seek help without fear of reprisal.

2. Work-Life Balance: Promote a healthy work-life balance by setting reasonable working hours, encouraging breaks, and discouraging excessive overtime. Avoid a culture of constant connectivity, allowing employees to disconnect after work hours.

3. Training and Education: Provide training to employees and managers about mental health awareness, recognizing signs of distress, and destigmatizing mental health challenges. Educated employees are more likely to be supportive of their colleagues.

4. Supportive Leadership: Foster a supportive leadership style where managers are approachable and understanding. Encourage open communication and create an atmosphere where employees feel comfortable discussing their mental health concerns.

5. Flexible Work Arrangements: Offer flexible work arrangements such as remote work, flexible hours, or compressed workweeks. This flexibility can help employees manage their mental health challenges effectively.

6. Anti-Discrimination Policies: Have clear anti-discrimination policies in place to protect employees with mental health conditions from discrimination. Promote a culture of acceptance and inclusion.

In Schools:

1. Mental Health Education: Integrate mental health education into the curriculum. Teach students about mental health, coping strategies, and the importance of seeking help when needed.

2. School Counseling Services: Provide access to school counselors who are trained to address mental health concerns. Ensure that students know about these services and feel comfortable using them.

3. Peer Support Programs: Establish peer support programs where students can talk to trained peers about their concerns. Peer support can often be more relatable and less intimidating for students.

4. Teacher Training: Provide teachers and staff with mental health training. Equip them with the knowledge and skills to recognize signs of mental distress in students and know how to respond appropriately.

5. Safe and Inclusive Environment: Foster a safe and inclusive school environment where bullying and discrimination are not tolerated. A positive social atmosphere can significantly impact students' mental well-being.

6. Parental Involvement: Involve parents in mental health initiatives. Educate parents about mental health, signs to look out for, and how to support their children's mental well-being at home.

By implementing these strategies, workplaces and schools can create environments where individuals feel supported, understood, and empowered to manage their mental health effectively.

The role of media in shaping perceptions of mental health

The media plays a significant role in shaping perceptions of mental health, often influencing public attitudes, beliefs, and behaviors. Here's how the media impacts our understanding of mental health:

1. Stigmatization vs. Awareness: Media can either reinforce mental health stigma by portraying individuals with mental illnesses in negative, sensationalized ways, or it can raise awareness by depicting their experiences accurately and with empathy. Responsible media coverage can help break down stereotypes and reduce stigma.

2. Portrayal of Mental Health Issues: Media, including movies, TV shows, and news stories, can influence how mental health issues are perceived. Sensationalized or inaccurate portrayals may lead to misunderstandings about specific disorders, symptoms, and treatments. Conversely, accurate and sensitive portrayals can enhance understanding.

3. Role Models: Positive portrayals of individuals living with mental health challenges, whether in movies, TV shows, or real-life stories, can provide role models for others, demonstrating that it's possible to live a fulfilling life despite mental health struggles.

4. Suicide Reporting: Media reporting on suicides requires careful handling. Irresponsible reporting can lead to copycat behavior, while responsible reporting can raise awareness about mental health issues and available support services without glamorizing self-harm.

5. Social Media Influence: Social media platforms can both positively and negatively impact mental health. On one hand, they can provide a sense of community and support for individuals dealing with mental health challenges. On the other hand, they can contribute to feelings of inadequacy, anxiety, and depression due to constant comparison with others.

6. News Media Impact: News stories about violent incidents involving individuals with mental illnesses can perpetuate the misconception that people with mental health issues are dangerous. In reality, individuals with mental health challenges are more likely to be victims of violence than perpetrators.

7. Advocacy and Awareness: Media can serve as a platform for mental health advocacy, helping organizations and individuals raise awareness, educate the public, and promote understanding about mental health issues and the importance of seeking help.

To promote positive perceptions of mental health, it's important for media outlets to portray mental health issues accurately, avoid sensationalism, and highlight stories of resilience and recovery. Additionally, media literacy programs can empower individuals to critically analyze media portrayals of mental health, fostering a more informed and compassionate society.

MENTAL HEALTH AND PHYSICAL HEALTH

The mind-body connection: How physical health influences mental well-being

The mind-body connection refers to the intricate relationship between your physical health and mental well-being. Engaging in regular physical activity has been shown to release endorphins, which are natural mood lifters, and reduce stress hormones, promoting a more positive outlook. Additionally, a balanced diet rich in nutrients can support brain function and emotional stability.

Furthermore, adequate sleep is crucial for both your body and mind. Lack of sleep can impair cognitive function and emotional regulation, leading to increased stress and anxiety. Chronic health conditions, pain, or inflammation in the body can also affect mental health, often leading to symptoms of depression and anxiety.

Overall, taking care of your physical health through exercise, nutrition, and proper rest plays a significant role in maintaining good mental well-being, highlighting the profound connection between the mind and body.

Exercise, nutrition, and their impact on mental health

Exercise and nutrition play vital roles in mental health. Regular physical activity is linked to the release of endorphins, which reduce feelings of pain and stress, leading to an improved mood and decreased anxiety. Exercise also promotes better sleep, increases self-esteem, and provides a sense of accomplishment.

Nutrition, on the other hand, directly affects brain function and mood. Consuming a balanced diet rich in essential nutrients such as omega-3 fatty acids, vitamins, and minerals supports brain health. For example, omega-3 fatty acids found in fish have been associated with reduced risk of depression and anxiety.

Additionally, maintaining stable blood sugar levels through proper nutrition helps regulate mood swings. Diets high in processed foods, sugar, and caffeine may contribute to increased feelings of anxiety and irritability.

In summary, regular exercise and a nutritious diet are powerful tools for promoting mental well-being. They can enhance mood, reduce stress, and contribute to overall emotional resilience. Integrating these healthy habits into daily life can significantly impact mental health positively.

Sleep and its role in maintaining mental and emotional balance.

Sleep plays a crucial role in maintaining mental and emotional balance. Quality sleep is essential for cognitive functions such as memory, attention, and decision-making. During sleep, the brain processes and consolidates memories, which is important for learning and emotional regulation.

Adequate sleep also regulates emotions. When you're well-rested, you are better able to manage stress, cope with challenges, and regulate your mood. Lack of sleep, on the other hand, can lead to increased irritability, difficulty concentrating, and heightened emotional responses. Chronic sleep deprivation has been linked to a higher risk of developing mood disorders like depression and anxiety.

Moreover, during the deep stages of sleep, the body repairs tissues, releases hormones that promote growth, and boosts immune function. This physical restoration is essential for overall well-being, including mental and emotional health.

Establishing a regular sleep schedule, creating a comfortable sleep environment, and practicing relaxation techniques can contribute to better sleep quality. Prioritizing sufficient sleep is essential for maintaining mental and emotional balance, improving resilience, and enhancing overall quality of life.

FUTURE TRENDS AND INNOVATIONS

Advancements in mental health research and treatment

Advancements in mental health research and treatment have been significant in recent years. Researchers have made substantial progress in understanding the biological, psychological, and social factors contributing to mental health disorders. One notable area of advancement is the exploration of neuroplasticity, which is the brain's ability to reorganize itself and form new neural connections. This understanding has led to innovative therapies and interventions.

Additionally, the field of psychopharmacology has seen the development of more targeted and effective medications with fewer side effects for various mental health conditions. Personalized medicine, where treatments are tailored to an individual's genetic makeup and specific symptoms, is becoming more prevalent, leading to more precise and efficient interventions.

Furthermore, advancements in psychotherapy techniques, such as cognitive-behavioral therapy (CBT), dialectical behavior therapy (DBT), and mindfulness-based therapies, have provided effective non-pharmacological options. Virtual reality therapy and online therapy platforms have also expanded access to mental health services, making treatment more accessible to a broader population.

Research in mental health has increasingly focused on prevention and early intervention strategies, aiming to identify and address mental health issues before they escalate. Public awareness campaigns and DE stigmatization efforts have contributed to a more open dialogue about mental health, encouraging individuals to seek help and support.

Overall, these advancements signify a more comprehensive and nuanced understanding of mental health conditions, leading to improved treatments, increased accessibility, and reduced stigma surrounding mental health issues.

The role of technology in mental health support (apps, online therapy, telemedicine)

Technology plays a crucial role in mental health support in various ways:

1. Accessibility: Technology provides accessible mental health resources to a global audience. People can access therapy, counseling, and self-help tools online, breaking down geographical barriers.

2. Anonymity and Privacy: Online platforms allow individuals to seek help anonymously, reducing the stigma associated with mental health issues. Many people find it easier to discuss their concerns in a digital format.

3. Convenience: Teletherapy and mental health apps offer convenient options for support. Individuals can schedule therapy sessions from the comfort of their homes, fitting it into their busy schedules more easily.

4. Immediate Support: Crisis helplines and text services offer immediate support to individuals in distress. Technology enables real-time communication with trained professionals, potentially preventing crises.

5. Personalized Interventions: AI-driven apps can offer personalized interventions based on users' responses and behaviors. These interventions can include mood tracking, coping strategies, and mental health exercises tailored to individual needs.

6. Education and Awareness: Technology facilitates the dissemination of mental health education and awareness. Online platforms, social media, and mobile apps provide information about mental health conditions, reducing misinformation and increasing understanding.

7. Monitoring and Prevention: Wearable devices and mobile apps can monitor physiological markers like heart rate and sleep patterns, providing insights into mental well-being. Early detection of irregularities can lead to timely interventions.

8. Therapeutic Tools: Virtual reality (VR) and augmented reality (AR) are used in exposure therapy and stress management. VR environments can simulate situations that trigger anxiety, allowing individuals to confront and manage their fears in a controlled setting.

9. Supportive Communities: Online forums and social media groups connect people facing similar mental health challenges. These communities provide a sense of belonging, understanding, and support.

10. Research and Data Analysis: Technology enables researchers to collect and analyze large datasets related to mental health. This data-driven approach helps in understanding patterns, improving treatments, and developing effective interventions.

It's important, however, to ensure that these technologies are developed and used responsibly, with a focus on user safety, data security, and ethical considerations. Additionally, combining technology with human empathy and professional expertise is essential for effective mental health support

Promising therapies on the horizon

Several promising therapies are on the horizon for mental health treatment, showing potential in improving outcomes for various mental health conditions:

1. Psychedelic-Assisted Therapy: Studies on psychedelics like psilocybin (found in certain mushrooms) and MDMA (commonly known as ecstasy) have shown promising results in treating conditions such as PTSD, depression, and anxiety disorders. These substances, when used in controlled therapeutic settings, may help individuals process traumatic experiences and alleviate symptoms.

2. Ketamine Therapy: Ketamine, traditionally used as an anesthetic, has gained attention for its rapid antidepressant effects. Ketamine infusion therapy is being explored as a treatment for severe depression, bipolar disorder, and PTSD.

3. Digital Therapeutics: Mobile apps and digital platforms offer evidence-based therapeutic interventions for mental health conditions. These digital therapeutics include cognitive-behavioral therapy (CBT) programs, mindfulness apps, and virtual reality treatments that can be accessed remotely.

4. Genetic and Precision Medicine: Advances in genetics are paving the way for personalized mental health treatments. Understanding an individual's genetic makeup can help tailor medications and therapies, increasing their efficacy and reducing side effects.

5. Neurostimulation Therapies: Non-invasive brain stimulation techniques like transcranial magnetic stimulation (TMS) and transcranial direct current stimulation (tDCS) are being explored for various mental health disorders, including depression and schizophrenia.

6. Microbiota Interventions: The gut-brain connection is an area of growing research. Manipulating the gut microbiota through probiotics and dietary interventions may have a positive impact on mental health conditions such as depression, anxiety, and autism spectrum disorders.

7. Artificial Intelligence (AI) in Therapy: AI-powered chatbots and virtual therapists are becoming more sophisticated, providing scalable and accessible mental health support. These technologies can offer immediate responses and personalized interventions based on users' input.

8. Integrative and Holistic Approaches: Therapies that integrate traditional mental health treatments with complementary approaches like acupuncture, yoga, and mindfulness are gaining popularity. These holistic approaches focus on the mind-body connection and overall well-being.

9. Brain-Computer Interfaces (BCIs): BCIs, which establish direct communication between the brain and external devices, are being researched for mental health applications. These interfaces have the potential to help individuals regulate brain activity and manage conditions like PTSD and anxiety disorders.

While these therapies hold promise, it's important to note that ongoing research and rigorous clinical trials are necessary to validate their safety and effectiveness. As our understanding of mental health deepens, these innovative therapies have the potential to revolutionize the field of mental health treatment.

CONCLUSION

Encouragement for seeking help and fostering a supportive environment.

Seeking help for mental health issues is a courageous step toward healing and well-being. It's a sign of strength, not weakness, to acknowledge your struggles and reach out for support. Remember that you don't have to face your challenges alone—there are compassionate professionals, friends, and family members who care about your well-being and want to help.

Fostering a supportive environment for mental health starts with open communication and empathy. Be kind to yourself and others. Listen without judgment and offer your support without reservation. Educate yourself and others about mental health to reduce stigma and increase understanding. Encourage those around you to seek help if they need it and be a source of encouragement throughout their journey.

Remember, asking for help is a powerful act of self-care. You deserve to live a life that is mentally, emotionally, and physically healthy. You are not alone, and there is hope and help available. Reach out, talk to someone you trust, and take the first step toward a brighter and healthier future

Final thoughts on the future of mental health awareness and advocacy

The future of mental health awareness and advocacy looks promising as society continues to prioritize mental well-being. Increased awareness has led to reduced stigma surrounding mental health issues, encouraging more open conversations and acceptance. In the years ahead:

1. Early Intervention: Early detection and intervention will be a focus, ensuring that individuals receive support before their mental health challenges escalate.

2. Digital Mental Health Services: Technology will continue to play a significant role, providing accessible and innovative mental health resources to a broader audience, especially in remote areas.

3. Holistic Approaches: There will be a shift toward holistic mental health care, acknowledging the interconnectedness of mental, emotional, and physical well-being. Integrative treatments that combine traditional and complementary therapies will become more prevalent.

4. Cultural Sensitivity: Mental health advocacy will be more culturally sensitive, recognizing and addressing the unique challenges faced by different communities. Culturally competent mental health services will become more widely available.

5. Global Collaboration: International collaboration will increase, enabling the sharing of knowledge, resources, and best practices to improve mental health support systems globally.

6. Education and Prevention: Schools and workplaces will prioritize mental health education and prevention programs, equipping individuals with the tools to maintain good mental health and support others.

7. Policy Changes: Advocacy efforts will lead to policy changes, ensuring mental health services are integrated into overall healthcare systems. Insurance coverage for mental health treatments will become more comprehensive and accessible.

8. DE stigmatization: Ongoing DE stigmatization efforts will lead to a society where mental health issues are viewed and treated like any other health condition, fostering understanding, empathy, and support for those affected.

By fostering a culture of empathy, understanding, and support, the future of mental health awareness and advocacy holds the promise of a world where everyone's mental health is valued, protected, and nurtured, leading to healthier, happier communities worldwide.